Hugh Oster

Steam Bathing

Health Benefits of Sweating

**HEALTH
HOUSE**
Publisher

Table of content

Introduction

During the 2015 Christmas holiday, we went the whole family to Costa Rica. I live in Montreal, where Canadian winters are hard on the body. Just before leaving I remember kids and wife complaining dry skin, runny nose, dry scalp and the week before I felt foggy brain.

We had a fantastic trip, I remember a day with 105 degrees Fahrenheit (41 °C) and near 100% humidity. Our ailments were all gone after two weeks spent there. Wow, back home I was thinking how can the weather do such a change to our condition. We live in houses with tempered conditions, but maybe too cold and dry for the body's natural heal power to cure and prevent many ailments.

I searched the Web to find how could we bring the Costa Rican climate back home... I looked at saunas, but It was too hot and dry to mimic this weather. Even wet saunas are still way to dry. Then I discovered steam bathing. Steam rooms are generally between 105 to 115 degrees Fahrenheit (41 to 46 °C) with 100% humidity. That was what I was looking for. I ran to the nearest home center and installed a steam shower device to our glass and tile shower. It took about a week part time to do the job; the steamer is in the basement and the shower is at the second floor. I also had to seal the top of the shower which was open. Since then we enjoy so much steam bathing that I searched all I could find about its health benefits. You will discover my finding in this book.

Many people in the 21st century turn to pharmaceutical drugs and conventional medicine to remedy their health problems, but overlook more natural alternatives that are equally as effective. For example, individuals who have insomnia might schedule an appointment with a doctor so they can get a prescription for sleeping pills like Ambien or Halcion. Highly stressed individuals might seek out a doctor for an anti-depressant like Prozac, to help reduce their stress-induced symptoms. Individuals who suffer from hypertension or migraines might also go to the doctor before researching other treatment options. Those with upper respiratory issues or sinus issues might visit a doctor's office before exploring a more natural approach.

Seeking out professional medical help is definitely a great way to stay healthy and find relief from chronic pain and other health concerns. However, many individuals have found relief in natural therapies (yoga, acupuncture, massage, supplements, breathing exercises, etc.). One of the best types of natural therapies out there is steam bathing. Steam bathing results in many health benefits, including: enhanced respiratory health, metabolism, weight loss, immunity, hair and skin health, and mental and physical relaxation.

But where did the use of steam bathing come from? What are the different types of steam treatments and steam baths? What exactly are the health benefits you can get? What are some easy ways to start incorporating steam bathing into your health routine?

It is the goal of this guide to equip you with the knowledge and tools you need to start living a healthier life by using steam baths.

The History of Steam Baths

Although many modern-day people flock to spas and gyms to make use of their saunas and/or steam bath rooms, they might not be aware of the ancient history of these practices. In reality, steam bathing was a common custom around the globe that has been around for hundreds of years.

The first steam bath rooms were thought to have originated in Egypt and Greece, as part of the royal palaces. We know more about the Greek steam baths, however, since their architectural remains were better preserved. Remains of Greek baths can be found in the cities of Athens, Olympia, and Corinth, as well as a few other cities. One of the earliest examples of a Greek steam bath room was the Queen's Bathroom in the palace of Knossos in Crete, which was built c. 1700 BC.

The Spartans invented the hot air bath, or what they deemed, laconica. These were more like a sauna than a steam bath, because they used a dry heat source. It is thought that the Greeks developed laconica baths for athletes, as a connecting space centered between the gym and the lecture hall. In their culture, health of the body was equally important as health of the mind.

Laconica baths started out as simple, rectangular structures about 4 meters wide and 20 meters long. The bath at Olympia is a great example of this preliminary design. As time went on, the baths became a bit more complex. Designers added extra basins for holding water; some even added swimming pools.

There were two different methods for heating laconica baths. One was the hot rock method, where people heated up rocks then transferred them to the bath area, to warm the room. The other method was to use coal burning fires, which would heat the surfaces of the room.

About 1500 years later, the Romans expanded upon the laconica bath room with their laconicum, and also added a steam bath room called the sudatorium. It was common for new emperors to win the people's favor by building thermae, which was a public bathing facility. These could cover the space of a few blocks and were similar to a modern-day gym structure, including cold and hot pools, exercise rooms, saunas, and steam rooms. They often had libraries and/or reading rooms connected to the steam room area. One of the largest thermae that we have remnants of is the Baths of Diocletian that had a 3000 persons capacity.

Besides thermae, the Romans also had smaller bath facilities called balneae, which could be either private or public. Steam bathing was a communal activity that most male Romans could easily afford. Later on, steam bathing for women was introduced. While some public baths were co-ed, these were usually frowned upon by refined, upper class members of society. Steam bathing became such a core social activity that according to a building catalogue dating to 354 AD, there were 952 recorded baths in the city of Rome alone. Roman baths were usually structured with three main rooms and some type of steam bath (sudatorium) or sauna (laconicum). Some Roman baths had both a laconicum and sudatorium. The three main rooms were the frigidarium, tepidarium, and caldarium, which ranged from cold to hot temperatures. More complex designs were added later on.

"Steam bathing became such a core social activity that according to a building catalogue dating to 354 AD, there were 952 recorded baths in the city of Rome alone."

Turkey is another culture which adopted the Roman practice of steam bathing, shortly after it took over some regions of the Roman Empire. Turkish citizens enjoyed using bath rooms called hammams, a spin-off of the Arabic word hamma which simply means "heating up." The Turks grew so fond of steam bathing, they even incorporated it into some of their social customs like bathing before a holiday or wedding, after a funeral, after having a baby. They even had a custom of a "guest bath" where old friends would be introduced to the new friend, in the social, communal setting of the hammam. Some hammams also provided massage services.

In North America, many Native Americans had sweat lodges where they bathed in preparation for certain festivals, like the Sun Dance ritual. Native Americans saw the sweat lodge as a spiritual place to renew mind and body, as well as to access spiritual entities for strength and wisdom. Some sweat lodge buildings were a dome shaped huts made from tree branches bound together with rawhide or grass ropes. Other sweat lodge buildings were wooden lodges made out of bark and planks. Ancient lodges were covered with animal hides, whereas modern sweat lodges are usually covered with tarps or blankets. This helps to hold in the heat and steam. The sweat lodge traditionally faced East, where they placed a sacred fire pit. This was also the direction where Father Sun, one of their key spiritual figures, rose each day. They considered the sweat lodge ceremony sacred because sweating symbolized spiritual cleanliness.

Other countries had their own form of steam bathing. The Japanese had sentos, the Koreans had jimjilbangs, the Russians had banyas, the Indians had temescals, the Finns had saunas, and the Germans had thermens. It would take a whole other book to relate the details, architectural layouts, and ceremonies of every steam bathing tradition around the globe. But hopefully, this gives you some idea of how widespread bathing practices have been since ancient times.

Steam Baths: Great for Detoxification of Internal Organs

Despite its ancient roots, the health benefits of steam bathing are still strongly relevant for the average contemporary individual as they were to people of ancient times. Modern day advocates for steam baths cite detoxification as one of the key benefits of this healthy practice. Why is detoxification so important for those desiring a healthy lifestyle? I mean, how can you tell if your body needs to be detoxified?

Detoxification is one controversial subject in recent days. Some advocate that only liver and kidneys eliminate toxins out of the body and that we should let them do their job. We are in a time of "no detox" trend vs the detox trend... Let's get back to science with an open mind and not fall into any of the side of the trends...

Chances are that if you live in the contemporary world, you likely do have some level of built up toxins in your body. From chemical food additives to toxic metals, from parabens and phthalates to petroleum and BPA, the modern-day environment has many sources of toxins that our bodies have access to simply by approximation. So how does contaminants enter the body.

"Detoxification is one controversial subject in recent days. Some advocate that only liver and kidneys eliminate toxins out of the body and that we should let them do their job."

Phthalates, for example, are a type of softener found in plastics, shampoos, laundry detergents, and some cosmetic products. Contact with this substance, results in the phthalates entering your bloodstream and negatively impacting your hormone levels. Some studies have shown that too much phthalate in the blood can impair testosterone production as well as interfere with reproductive development. Other health experts link phthalates to conditions like obesity, autism, ADHD, breast cancer, and asthma.

BPA is a substance found in plastic containers and water bottles. It is linked to early onset puberty, infertility, and heart disease in both genders. Other research claims that BPA can cause negative effects on the brain, specifically by interfering with the Kcc2 gene, which in turn, results in central nervous system damage.

Some toxic chemicals are actually carcinogens that are surprisingly common in cosmetic products. BHA, BHT, petrolatum, sodium laureth sulfate, and coal tar dyes (which are often indicated on the label as colors, CI followed by a five-digit number). Other substances in cosmetics release formaldehyde: imidazolidinyl urea, diazolidinyl urea, methenamine, DMDM hydantoin, and quarternium-15. Siloxane ingredients (indicated by –methicone or –siloxane, on the ingredients list) have been shown to interfere with the reproductive and endocrine systems.

Besides these common sources of chemicals, you must also consider other common environmental chemicals that the average person encounters on a daily basis. Pollution from car exhaust and coal-fired power plants; pesticides used in agriculture and for personal lawn and garden care; industrial chemicals that seep into the air from processing plants and chemical manufacturers; chemicals found in food packaging, furniture, and construction materials. Health experts link environmental toxics with contributing to cancer, Alzheimer's, autism, a weakened immune system, cardiovascular disease, and fibromyalgia.

So exactly what happens to these chemicals when they come in contact with your skin? The main way that toxins enter the body is through the body's largest organ, the skin. It's hard to think of your skin as an actual organ, however, the average adult has 22 square feet of skin, which translates to 8 pounds. Once toxins hit the skin, they are absorbed into the bloodstream and retained in intercellular fluid and fat cells. Hundreds of chemicals have been found in skin tissue. Most of the toxins are concentrated in the liver and blood.

"It's hard to think of your skin as an actual organ, however, the average adult has 22 square feet of skin, which translates to 8 pounds"

Exactly how do steam baths get rid of toxins in your body? The use of steam baths for personal health is sometimes referred to as hyperthermic therapy (or sweat therapy). Steam baths make your body sweat. This, in turn, opens up skin pores to release toxins, dirt, and debris from the skin. Steam bathing is particularly beneficial and safe practice for those suffering from kidney or liver problems. In fact, only 20 minutes or less of steam bathing will remove one day's worth of toxins and sweat from your body. Other statistics claim that the heat from the steam opens up 2.6 million sweat glands in your skin. With just one steam bath, your body eliminates as much as 30% of bodily waste.

Studies have confirmed the unique role that sweating plays in detoxifying the human body. In 2011, Archives of Environmental and Contamination Toxicology published a study confirming that the sweat process might be a better indicator of toxin concentration in an individual than analyzing urine and blood samples. "Toxic elements were found to differing degrees in each of blood, urine, and sweat. [...] Many toxic elements appeared to be preferentially excreted through sweat" (Stephen J Genuis, Detlef Birkholz, Ilia Rodushkin, Sanjay Beesoon)[i].

Despite the medical advances of the 21st century, it is interesting how frequently many conventional doctors overlook environmental exposure as a factor in their patients' health. According to Sayer Ji, founder of GreenMedInfo.com, some toxins and heavy metals do not show up on the urine or blood analysis results. Instead, they appear only on the sweat sample analysis. He states: "The obvious alternative method - identify and remove the poisons - isn't even on the table, unless the practitioner happens to be aware of natural, integrative or functional medical principles and has the courage to go against the FDA-approved and liability-shielding grain to employ them."

The 2011 report had some specific findings that highlight the important role that sweat plays in eliminating toxins and heavy metals from the body. For instance, higher concentration of cadmium was found in sweat rather than in blood. Another finding was that individuals who regularly used saunas had healthier mercury levels. There was a correlation between individuals with high body burden (or higher exposure to environmental toxins) and the presence of a high concentration of toxins in that individual's sweat. The study also found that the daily sweat process eliminates just as much or even more toxins as the urinary process does.

In 2012, the University of Alberta's Faculty of Medicine published two reports that proved how effective the sweat process is in eliminating BPA and phthalates. Researchers found BPA concentrations in some individuals' sweat samples, even if their urine and blood samples showed no BPA levels. When researchers tested for phthalate concentration, some individuals showed phthalate concentration in their sweat but not in their blood samples. Still other individuals had twice as much phthalate concentration in their sweat than in their urine.

Steam baths work better at detoxifying the body than using a sauna. In steam bathing, the body retains heat for a longer period, so you can get better results in less time; whereas in a sauna, you'd have to be in there for twice as long and the results wouldn't be as great.

The skin with its size and functions allow to expel lots of substances out of the body. You need to wash then out after sweating with soap and water if you want to prevent the skin to reabsorb them.

Benefits to Your Respiratory System

One of the major benefits of steam bathing are for your respiratory system. Steam bathing soothes inflamed throat and/or nasal passages, which makes it great therapy if you have a cold, the flu, asthma, allergies, sinusitis, or bronchitis. It can minimize coughing because it soothes your body's muscles. It can also act as an expectorant because it increases your body's secretions, which results in clearer secretions. Steam also moistens air passages and loosens mucus so blowing your noise and coughing are more productive in clearing your respiratory system.

Steam bathing has great benefits for people with lung disease. Steam therapy helps increase the total lung volume. This in turn aids the lungs' capacity to more easily inhale and exhale air. People with respiratory diseases should definitely consider using steam therapy to help combat their symptoms. It has proven useful for anyone with COPD (Chronic obstructive pulmonary disease)[ii], which includes the subcategories of chronic bronchitis, emphysema, and asthma.

For patients with bronchitis, some health experts recommend steam therapy with eucalyptus oil or other essential oils like peppermint, frankincense, or lavender. These oils enhance the warm steam's soothing properties to help your sinuses, bronchial passages, and lungs. They will also enhance the steam's expectorant properties, to thin mucous and trigger more productive coughing.

For many patients with asthma, steam rooms have helped minimize their symptoms where other treatments have failed. The warm moisture of the steam room can open up the lungs and bronchial tubes and relax the muscles. However, some doctors caution against steam rooms for certain types of asthma. **For instance, some people's symptoms worsen in high-humidity conditions, while others are improved. So, if you have asthma, make sure to consult with a doctor before using steam rooms.**

Besides bronchitis and asthma, steam therapy might have beneficial effects for soothing emphysema symptoms. But it varies from person to person. Some people choke on the steam from a hot shower while others breathe easier after taking steam baths. Emphysema is often caused by smoking, however, sometimes it can be caused by environmental chemicals or genetics. Patients with emphysema have trouble breathing or working out for long periods because the tiny air sacs in their lungs become inflamed and often damaged. Coughing and breathlessness are two primary symptoms of this disease. **Very cold, hot, or dry air can trigger a COPD (Chronic obstructive pulmonary disease) flare-up. So make sure to consult your doctor if you have COPD before using steam bathing.**

"During winter months, daily steam bathing is a good way to PREVENT cold and flu, particularly for those who are prone to respiratory track condition."

Steam bathing is also beneficial for minimizing symptoms of allergies and sinusitis. Steam therapy can soothe nasal and throat passages, while clearing out mucus and making it easier to breathe. Steam can also help with vocal hoarseness because it moisturizes the throat and vocal chords, the root cause of hoarseness. Many people with chronic allergies and/or sinusitis have found relief through alternative therapies like steam therapy, instead of pursuing more severe medical treatments like using antibiotics or steroids or undergoing sinus surgery.

For individuals with allergies or sinusitis, steam inhalations not only have anti-microbial properties, but they minimize inflammation and clear out the sinuses. Steam is effective particularly with sinus infections considering that the root cause of sinus infections are bacteria and (in some cases) molds and/or viruses. Health experts recommend doing an at-home steam treatment 2-4 times each day. Again, if you don't have a steam shower at home, you can boil water via microwave or stove, then pour it in a bowl and cover your head with a towel. Hold your face over the bowl for 10 minutes. Thought, it may not have the intensity a steam bath would provide.

Others have experienced relief by incorporating essential oils into their steam treatment, like eucalyptus, rosemary, tea tree, or myrtle oil. Simply add 2-3 drops each of these oils to your water before covering your head and putting your face over the bowl of water. Another steam inhalation "recipe" is to use two drops each of peppermint, eucalyptus, and lavender oil. You can also add handfuls of dried herbs (bergamot and thyme) to the hot water. Besides herbs and essential oils, apple cider vinegar is another ingredient that some people add to their hot water. Not only does apple cider vinegar have anti-inflammatory properties, its 5-6% concentration of acetic acid kills bacteria and reduces infection in your nasal and sinus passages.

Consult the book section about Enhancing the **Effects of Steam Bathing: Essential Oils** for more "recipe".

During winter months, daily steam bathing is a good way to PREVENT cold and flu, particularly for those who are prone to respiratory track condition.

Benefits to Your Skin and Hair

Skin

We saw how the skin can act as an organ for your body, but steam bathing provides great benefits for your skin itself. For one thing, it can help clear up acne and acne related conditions. Steam bathing acts as an enzymatic exfoliator that

helps to unclog pores from dirt and sebum that can trigger acne. Steam bathing is also useful for getting rid of blackheads and whiteheads, since clogged pores are the root cause of this skin condition. The steam opens up skin pores, so that the individual can extract the blackheads and whiteheads. Clean pores will help prevent future blackheads and whiteheads from forming.

Steam bathing is also useful for glowing skin and minimizing the appearance of wrinkles. Steam helps remove dead skin cells to reveal the newer, more luminous skin underneath. Wrinkles are common especially after you turn 30. Steam bathing can help fight the aging process because it heats the skin and stimulates blood circulation. It also eliminates toxins and seals in moisture, which makes your skin look younger and smoother.

Steam is also great for dry skin sufferers. Steam rooms have a 100% humidity level, which makes them moisturizing for people with dry skin. The moisture in the steam hydrates the skin's top layers. Also, the heat of the steam will raise the skin's temperature will triggers increased circulation. If you have dry skin, make sure to put on some sort of lotion or moisturizer after a steam bath; this will help seal in the moisture gained from the steam and prevent the skin from drying out after the bath.

Steam bathing can also be great for people with dandruff. Using a steam room twice a week for just ten minutes can greatly minimize the appearance of dandruff. This is because dandruff is often caused by dry scalp conditions, a symptom which steam excels at eradicating.

If your goal is to use stream treatment for all of your skin, the steam room or using an at-home steam shower will be your best bet. If your goal is to target the skin on your face and you don't have steam equipment at home, the easiest way to do this is to boil some hot water, put it in a bowl, cover your head and face with a towel and hold your head over the bowl, so your face soaks in the steam. Keep your head over the bowl for about 10 minutes to gain maximum benefits.

Exfoliation of dry skin is easy while steam bathing. Just after steam showering I usually gently rub dry skin patches with a wet washcloth and rinse. This removes all dead skin cells.

Hair

Steam bathing is also beneficial to hair health. It can be moisturizing especially for naturally curly or coarse hair. Steaming hair has four main benefits: it lifts the hair cuticle, defines curls and increases volume, boosts strength and elasticity, and helps prevent the hair from getting "hygral fatigue." Lifting the cuticle is great for hair because it allows more moisture and other nourishing hair product ingredients to penetrate the hair follicle. Steam bathing will also define curls, add volume, and make curly/coarse hair strands more resistant to breakage. People with naturally curly or coarse hair also have to deal with the concern of "hygral fatigue" to their hair. Hygral fatigue happens when hair is washed too frequently and/or if the hair is receiving too much moisture on a regular basis. This is because when the hair absorbs water, the cuticle expands then rapidly contracts, when the cuticle dries out. For non-curly and/or fine hair, that process is usually not a problem. But for naturally curly or coarse hair, this expansion and contraction process can cause cracked or frayed hair cuticles which causes the overall hair to be drier and brittle. Hair experts state that steam treatments combined with hair oil treatment (like coconut oil or some other natural oil) is the best way to maintain curly/coarse hair, between washes.

There are several ways to steam your hair directly, besides using a steam room:

Steam Tools

There are quite a few tools made specifically for steaming your hair. Check out Amazon or your local retail store's hair care section for table top and/or handheld steaming tools. Since these can be a bit pricey for some budgets, purchasing a deep conditioning heat cap can be a more affordable option. These caps typically have an attached cord that you plug into an electrical outlet, to control the heat level of the cap. Hair experts recommend using a heat cap about 3 times a week, for about 20-30 minutes each session.

Hot Towel Method

Moisten a towel in water, then heat it up for 2 minutes (in the microwave). Wrap the towel around your hair in a turban style—or use a shower cap, to trap the moisture and heat. Blow dry your covered hair with a hair dryer for at least 10 minutes. You can use this method before your normal shampoo and conditioning routine, or else every now and then to improve your hair's receptivity to hair products and moisturizers.

Oil Treatment, Then Hot Towel Method

Giving your hair an oil treatment before using the hot towel method can enhance the benefits of the steam on your hair. This is especially useful if your hair is dry and/or damaged. 2-4 times a month, try massaging coconut oil onto your scalp for 5-10 minutes (or use another type of hair health related oil, like argan or jojoba oil). Then use the hot towel steam method.

Steam treatments are healthy for your hair because they also enhance hair growth. The heat from a steam treatment warms your scalp, which stimulates blood flow. Increased blood flow at your scalp stimulates hair growth. Another way that steam boosts hair growth is because it clears blocked pores in your scalp. Hair follicles can only grow if the scalp's pores are clear, open, and free of toxins, dirt, and oils.

Other Health Benefits

Weight loss

Steam bathing provides a whole range of other health benefits, as well. For one thing, it enhances weight loss by boosting your metabolism and reducing water retention. Both built up toxins and water play a significant role in your overall body weight. Steam bathing lowers your body weight by making your body sweat, which eliminates impurities, sodium and water that your body has been accumulating and storing as extra pounds.

In comparison from being inactive, steam bathing increase blood circulation, increase your metabolism and activate sweat glands (2.6 million), which all contribute to weight loss. Some water will be rehydrate the body by drinking, but weigh loss comes from less sodium so less water retention, fat burned from energy used and ultimately less minerals and toxins.

Unintentional weight loss

On the other hand, people suffering long date unintentional weight loss have note weight gain after practicing steam bathing on regular basis. Unintentional weight loss usually comes from body dysfunctions. From mental conditions to organs, steam bathing may help regain weight by its broad action.

Steam bathing is useful for those with weak immune systems or individuals who feel like they are coming down with a cold. The steam room increases the body's internal temperature to 101 degrees Fahrenheit (39 °C), similar to that of a fever. The high temperature itself is enough to help kill viruses, bacteria, and other toxins accumulated in your body because they cannot withstand high heat.

The toxins that exit your body from the sweat are another way to rebuild your immune system's defenses against illness. In addition, this high temperature also triggers white blood cell production, another main way that your body destroys bacteria and viruses.

Headaches

Studies show that steam bathing can help individuals who suffer from frequent migraines or tension headaches. Once again, this is due to your body sweating, then releasing endorphins. Health experts recommend using steam therapy as soon as you start to feel a migraine coming on. But, steam bathing can be especially helpful if the headaches are related to sinus pressure and/or allergies. The steam will help to loosen mucus from the sinus passages and lessen the pressure an individual feel in their temples and face.[iii]

Vocal strain

Another perk of steam bathing is that it minimizes vocal strain and hoarseness. This is useful not just for individuals who experience vocal hoarseness in the winter, when indoor heaters dry the air of moisture, but also for professional singers. For singers, their vocal chords are their main instrument that they use for their job. Over performing as well as low-humidity environments can take its toll on the voice. Celine Dion sings at The Colosseum at Caesars Palace were stage is maintained at 55% humidity to provide a voice-soothing environment. Steam therapy moisturizes sinus membranes, which imparts moisture to the air before it hits the lungs. Also, steam therapy moisturizes the vocal chords which results in a steady vocal tone and supple vocal chords[iv]. Health experts recommend that professional singers use a steam therapy at least twice a day, like in the morning and in evening. During heavy performance seasons, health experts recommend doing steam therapy as often as four times a day.

> *" Celine Dion sings at The Colosseum at Caesars Palace were stage is maintain at 55% humidity to provide a voice-soothing environment."*

Minor health issues and socialize

Besides helping different health issues, steam bathing can also improve less serious health issues. For example, many people claim that steam bathing helps an individual recover from a hangover faster. Alcohol triggers toxin production in the pancreas, which can lead to conditions like pancreatitis. Sweating helps purge the body of toxins in general, which include the toxins associated with the alcohol consumption.

Other individuals claim that steam therapy helps them to get a closer shave and minimize the appearance of cellulite. Thus, steam bathing can minimize the use women does of cellulite fighting scrubs, lotions, and supplements.

Still others advocate steam bathing because it is a great way to socialize. Maybe the Greeks and Romans had it right when they started steam rooms in the first place, as a place for dialoguing with other citizens about personal and intellectual matters. In today's hurried world of over-packed schedules, going to a steam room with some friends can be a great way to destress, improve your health, and build relationships at the same time.

Steam Bathing for Athletes

Steam bathing is especially beneficial for athletes, particularly those in endurance related sports. The main way that steam therapy works for athletes is that it increases their core temperature for short intervals of time. Steam bathing helps increase an athlete's physical stamina because it helps condition their body to higher core temperatures, which makes it easier for their body to function when performing whatever sport they do. The Journal of Science in Medicine and Sport published a 2007 study[v] showing that higher plasma and red blood cell volume in runners who had a post-workout steam bath, compared to runners who did not. Some doctors claim that steam bathing can even trigger new growth in brain cells.

Heat treatments like steam bathing combined with exercise can help athletes enhance their muscle growth. The main way it does this is by triggering the body to produce more HGH, or human growth hormone. HGH is a biochemical that is essential for growing and maintaining muscle mass. This is particularly important after the age of 30, the point where HGH levels start to decrease significantly. An additional way that steam bathing catalyzes muscle growth is by releasing HSPs, or heat shock proteins. HSPs both prevent and repair damaged proteins in the body, which in turn, impacts muscle growth and maintenance.

"This is particularly important after the age of 30, the point where HGH levels start to decrease significantly. An additional way

that steam bathing catalyzes muscle growth is by releasing HSPs, or heat shock proteins"

According to one study published in 2007 by the Department of Applied Physiology and Kinesiology, University of Florida, rats exposed to intervals of heat therapy had 30% more muscle regrowth than the rats that were not exposed[vi]. Other research indicates that the elevation of HSPs in the body can last up to 48 hours after the heat therapy. When athletes combine a heat therapy like steam bathing with exercise, they maximize their body's HSP level, which in turn, maximizes their muscle mass.

Yet another way that steam therapy can benefit athletes is that it boosts the brain's production of neurotrophic factors like BDNF (brain-derived neurotrophic factor). BDNF helps both your brain and muscles. BDNF protects neuro-motor degradation, which helps prevent muscle atrophy. It also helps your brain by preventing and reducing brain degeneration.

Steam therapy also benefits the brain because it increases prolactin, norepinephrine, and endorphins. Prolactin is in charge of myelin growth, which helps the brain repair nerve cell damage and to function at high speed. During exercise and steam therapy use, an individual's norepinephrine levels increase 2-4 times. Norepinephrine increases mental clarity and focus needed for athletic performance. Studies have proven that the temperature of steam bathing alone has positive results on athletes, because it raises the body's endorphin level. So instead of a "runner's high," athletes who steam bath can get a "steam bathing high."

Steam bathing is also great for speeding muscle recovery. Athletes frequently experience DOMS (delayed onset muscle soreness) as a result of over training in the weight room. DOMS happens because muscle training literally "rips" the muscle tissue. These "rips" are actually micro-trauma lesions. DOMS symptoms usually show up 24-72 hours after an athlete's workout. Many athletes use steam therapy to reduce toxins and lactic acids that accumulate in their muscles during workouts. The steam therapy triggers an increase of endorphins, which helps reduce the body's sensation of pain associated with DOMS. The heat from the steam also relaxes the muscles, which helps the muscle tissue to heal faster.

Steam therapy can also help combat the frequent injuries that athletes encounter on the job by shortening their recovery time. When doctors prescribe an injured athlete a recovery plan, the plan usually has some component that will help the athlete minimize protein breakdown in their muscle tissue. As we said before, the heat associated with steam therapy can help reduce muscular atrophy. It also lowers the production of free radicals, which is common in muscle tissue when an athlete gets injured and takes a break from their usual workout routine.

Another way steam therapy can help injury recovery is that it boosts muscle tissue regrowth and minimizes the oxidation rates in the body. Steam therapy speeds up the healing process in another way: by expanding blood vessels, which increases blood circulation. Increased circulation means that more oxygen and nutrients in the blood can reach damaged muscle tissue and/or joints. This helps curb the athlete's pain and speeds the muscle/joint repair from the injury.

Besides repairing the actual muscle tissue and minimizing pain sensations, steam bathing can also increase an athlete's flexibility. Stretching is an essential part of any athlete's routine. It helps minimize joint and muscle injury while training and competing. As mentioned before, the heat from the steam helps to relax the muscle tissues in the body. It is way easier to stretch relaxed muscles than tense muscles. In fact, Auburn University Montgomery Kinesiology Laboratory did a study that found a 205% increase in flexibility in individuals who stretched in a heat therapy room compared to individuals that stretched outside of a heat therapy room. Athletes who follow up their workout routines with a steam bath session minimize their risk for damaging their muscle tissue when they perform their post-workout stretches.

Mental Health Benefits

Although steam bathing has many perks for your body, it can also enhance your mental health, as well. For one thing, steam bathing can help to clear your mind and relieve stress. The steam room atmosphere is usually quiet and minimalistic. Also, sweating helps calm the body, relax the muscles, and release endorphins which will enhance a calm state of mind. Steam bathing can be especially helpful for individuals who suffer from tension headaches caused from high stress circumstances at work or at home.

Steam bathing is also valuable for individuals who struggle with insomnia. Many people who are low on sleep resort to sleeping pills to keep them on a regular sleep schedule. Steam bathing is a natural way to help get a good night's sleep without using these drugs. Health experts recommend doing a 20-minutes steam room session about two hours before bedtime. Doing steam bathing before bed has a similar effect as a workout, because it increases the body's core temperature and boosts circulation. The steam and heat will relax your body physically, which in turn, will help you to fall asleep more quickly. Also, steam therapy has been proven to increase the amount of REM sleep that your body gets.

Steam bathing is also a great way to reduce anxiety and depression symptoms. As mentioned before, the sweat that a steam room triggers releases endorphin. David Muzina, MD from the Cleveland Clinic Center for Mood Disorders Treatment and Research, states that when the body sweats it "stimulates the release of many of the brain chemicals thought to be in low supply when someone is battling depression." Sweating releases good brain chemicals like endorphins, neurotransmitters, and endocannabinoids, which minimize sensations of pain and promote an overall feeling of positive wellbeing (both mentally and physically). The sweat induced by a steam room can also help depression by reducing the chemicals in your immune system that can worsen depression.

Besides depression, those who suffer from anxiety should try steam bathing, as well. The temperature of a steam bath is enough to help calm the mind and body, because it raises your internal body temperature. When you leave the steam room, your body experiences a cool down, which relaxes you mentally and physically. There is definitely a link between having a calm, relaxed body and having a calm, relaxed mental state. Individuals who steam bath claim to have calmer thoughts and an overall sense of peace and positive energy, after they do a steam therapy session.

Steam bathing with friends has an added benefit to mental health. Not only does socializing provide a positive distraction from focusing on anxious thoughts, it has been scientifically proven to boost oxytocin production in the body. Often called "the pleasure hormone," oxytocin promotes an overall feeling of happiness and greatly reduces both stress and anxiety in the body.

Basic Types of Installation

There are many ways to steam bath. Some gyms offer steam room facilities as part of their membership benefits. Spas are another common place to find steam rooms and/or steam therapy facilities. Other people prefer to do steam bathing at home.

For those who wish to do steam bathing at home, there are two main options to pick from when choosing which type of steam bath or room to install: a steam room and a steam shower. A steam room is just that: a room equipped and set aside in your house for use as a steam room. A steam shower, on the other hand, is simply a shower equipped with a steam bath function.

There are pros and cons for each type. For example, if you do not have much space in your house, a steam shower might be your best option. You also want to consider how many people will use the steam shower/room and whether they want to do it alone or with another member of the house. For only one person, a steam shower is usually the best option. For more people, a steam room can be the better option since it has the capacity for two or more people. Another factor to consider is convenience. Some individuals find a steam shower more convenient since it's just an added function to their main shower. A steam room is often more inconvenient, since (depending on your house's layout) it is usually not part of your bathroom, but in a separate, more remote location in your house. A more remote location means it will be harder to access.

Guidelines for installing a steam room

- Pay attention to the manufacturer's instructions when installing a steam room.
- Make sure the steam room is properly sealed and insulated. This will prevent heat from escaping the steam room and protect any adjacent walls, ceilings, and flooring from water damage.
- Pick the right type of generator. This will vary on the size of the steam room. Besides the size of your steam room, know what your budget is. Like with any home improvement tools and equipment, steam room generators have a wide price range.
- Another thing to consider is what material your steam room is made out of. Each type of material will require a specific type of generator. A porcelain tiled steam room will need a bigger generator than a marble or fiberglass steam room because the material type influence greatly the energy needed to heat the room, as if adjacent to an exterior wall.
- Finally make sure to have access to shower yourself inside or nearby the steam room.

Guidelines for installing a steam shower

- Make sure your room is well sealed and insulated, to both contain the steam shower's heat and prevent water damage to any adjacent walls, ceilings, and flooring.
- Ensure that the water drains efficiently, to prevent mildew and/or water damage to the shower.

- Make sure the shower doors seal in the steam. You might also want to waterproof plaster or sheet-rock that is adjacent to the shower. Another suggestion is to install a plastic layer under the shower, to act as a steam barrier.
- Yet another factor to consider is installing the shower so that condensation does not drip directly onto the people using the shower.

Portable steam bath

Yet another option is to purchase a portable steam bath or "cabinet." If you go with this option, please follow these guidelines:

- Follow manufacturer instructions for your portable steam bath or cabinet.
- Put the portable steam bath in a room that is properly sealed and insulated.
- Make sure to have an appropriate power outlet to hook up to.

Enhancing the Effects of Steam Bathing: Essential Oils

Although steam showers and baths are great ways to incorporate steam therapy into your life, these additions to your home can be expensive. There are many ways to incorporate steam therapy into your life without having to reconfigure your house.

For example, some individuals boil water in a pot on the stove, then put their face over the pot and cover their head with a towel, to help create a greenhouse effect. This is a great way to help clear your sinuses, alleviate headaches, or minimize skin pores on your face. 10 minutes is a sufficient amount of time to do this facial steaming session.

Another easy way to do your own steam therapy is to fill up your normal bath tub with hot water (as hot as you can comfortably stand). Then add Epsom salts or essential oils like eucalyptus or lavender to your bath, depending on which health concern you are trying to target (sore muscles, headache, insomnia, etc.).

Many individuals incorporate herbs and/or essential oils into their steam bathing practices to maximize the soothing effects of steam bathing. There are many different "recipes" of therapeutic ingredients you can add to your at-home steam bath. Here are just some of them:

Epsom Salt for General Detoxification

Another name for Epsom salt is magnesium sulfate. Epsom salt has a wide variety of health perks. It can flush toxins from your body; improve nutrient absorption; relieve stress, migraine headaches, and insomnia; enhance your mental clarity and focus; minimize muscle cramps and inflammation; build up brain tissue, mucin proteins, and joint protein; prevent blood clots and hardened arteries; and boost oxygen use.

Steam Bath Recipe:

Start with ¼ cup Epsom salt. You can gradually increase this portion to 2 cups Epsom salt per bath. Add to hot bath water. Soak for 10-20 minutes.

Ginger for Inflamed Muscles and Indigestion

This spicy root is useful to add to steam baths because of its detoxifying properties. Ginger has a high concentration of the anti-inflammatory and anti-spasmodic components called gingerol and shoga. Ginger is a great ingredient to help cleanse the liver, colon, and organs of toxins. It can also neutralize acids in the digestive system, which in turn, relieves symptoms like indigestion, bloating, and upset stomach.

Steam Bath Recipe:

Boil a pot of water on the stove and put ½ inch slice of ginger root into the water. Turn off the heat and let stand for 30 minutes. Take out the ginger, then add this boiling water to your bath water. Soak for 10-20 minutes.

Eucalyptus for Sinus Headaches

Eucalyptus oil is very popular for minimizing sinusitis and alleviating sinus headaches. This oil is known for its anti-inflammatory, antifungal, antibacterial, antimicrobial, antiviral, and decongestant properties. Eucalyptus oil treatment is especially beneficial for helping individuals recover faster from non-bacterial sinusitis.

Steam Bath Recipe:

Add the following to your hot bath water: 10 drops Sesame Seed Oil, 5 drops Eucalyptus oil, 1 tbsp Sesame Seed Oil. Soak for 10-20 minutes.

Lemon for Enhanced Immunity and Energy

Lemon oil is great for energizing the body and boosting the immune system due to its high vitamin concentration. It is also useful for targeting asthma, insomnia, hair and skin conditions, fatigue, stress disorders, fever and infections.

Steam Bath Recipe:

Add the following to your hot bath water: 5 drops Lemon essential oil, 5 drops Lemon Eucalyptus oil, 2 drops Tea Tree oil, 2 drops Pine Needle oil, 2 tbsp coconut oil. Soak for 10-20 minutes.

Peppermint for Muscle and Joint Soreness

Peppermint oil is great for soothing sore joints and muscles, as well as soothing your stomach. It also acts as an antimicrobial. Using this oil in a steam bath can help improve mental focus, relieve headaches, and clear the respiratory system.

Steam Bath Recipe:

Add the following to your hot bath water: 5 drops citrus oil, 5 drops peppermint oil, 2 drops clove oil, 1 tbsp jojoba oil. Soak for 10-20 minutes.

Lavender for Insomnia

Lavender oil is great for insomnia. Researchers at Britain's University of Southampton performed a study on 10 adults. Half the participants slept in a lavender scented room and the other half slept in an unscented room. The participants who slept in the lavender scented room reported a 20% increase in the quality of their sleep, compared to the other participants.

Steam Bath Recipe:

Add the following to your hot bath water: 10 drops Lavender essential oil, 6 drops Chamomile essential oil, 1 tbsp jojoba oil, 2-3 tbsp sea salt. Soak for 10-20 minutes.

Frankincense for Anxiety

Frankincense oil is great for reducing anxiety symptoms. It has a sedative effect on the body, reducing blood pressure and clearing respiratory pathways.

Steam Bath Recipe:

Add the following to your hot bath water: 10 drops Frankincense essential oil, 10 drops Rose essential oil, 2-3 tbsp sea salt, 2 tbsp coconut oil. Soak for 10-20 minutes.

Bergamot for Stress, Anxiety, or Depression

Bergamot oil is known for its anti-inflammatory, antibacterial, antispasmodic, and anti-infectious properties. It is also great for minimizing symptoms of stress and anxiety because it acts as a sedative and relaxant. Bergamot is also a natural anti-depressant that can greatly minimize depression symptoms.

Grapefruit for Detoxification, Arthritis, or Menstrual Cramps

Grapefruit oil is a less common essential oil, but it has great perks. Not only is it a great detoxifier, but it can help reduce symptoms of acne, exhaustion, arthritis, rheumatism, menstrual cramps, stiffness and stress.

Steam Bath Recipe:

Add 15 drops of grapefruit essential oil to your hot bath water. Soak for 10-20 minutes.

Rosemary for Enhanced Memory and Alzheimer's Prevention

Ancient Greek scholars wore rosemary on their heads when taking tests, to boost their memory. Besides enhanced memory, rosemary oil can help prevent and treat symptoms of Alzheimer's. Psychogeriatrics published a study featuring 28 elderly participants with dementia (17 of these had Alzheimer's). Rosemary was one of the key oils incorporated into the experiment. The study found that individuals experienced an improved sense of orientation after the exposure to rosemary and a few other essential oils.

Steam Bath Recipe:

Add 2 tbsp olive oil and 10 drops Rosemary essential oil to your hot bath water. Soak for 10-20 minutes.

Proper Use of Steam Baths

Toxins mixes with sweat. In order to prevent reabsorption of toxins, right after sweating, shower and clean the body with soap.

Whatever type of steam room, shower or bath that you decide to use, there are some common safety rules to follow to maximize your health benefits and reduce health risks. The appropriate temperature of a steam room ranges from 105 to 115 degrees Fahrenheit (41 to 46 °C). Most health experts claim to spend no more than 15-20 minutes in a steam room. When in a steam room, make sure to follow these basic rules:

- Make sure to drink plenty of water before and after being in the steam room, to prevent dehydration.
- Wear light clothing when going into the steam room, to avoid overheating.
- Avoid eating right before steam bathing. This is because the steam room affects your body's digestion and blood circulation. A good rule of thumb is to cut off food an hour before the time you plan on steam bathing.
- Avoid all alcoholic beverages before and after steam bathing.
- Don't go over the 15-20 minutes recommended time limit.
- If you feel dizzy or nauseous, leave the steam room or stop your at-home steam session.

Although steam bathing is beneficial for many individuals, there are some individuals who should not use steam bathing. If you have rosacea, high blood pressure, or a heart condition, experts recommend avoiding steam therapy treatments. Also, if you are pregnant and/or nursing, steam bathing is not recommended. Consult your doctor before using steam bathing.

Conclusion

Whether used with essential oils, or on its own, steam bathing is definitely an effective, natural treatment for many health conditions. From anxiety and depression to muscle/joint soreness, steam bathing has a wide spectrum of benefits to offer every individual who adopts this healthy practice. The wide variety of steam therapies and the different structures of steam baths make steam bathing accessible and cost-efficient to most people. We hope that this guide has equipped you with the information you need to start tapping into the potent perks of steam bathing.

Steam Bathing by Hugh Oster

Published by Health House Publisher

© 2017 Health House Publisher

References

[i] Genuis SJ, Birkholz D, Rodushkin I, Beesoon S. (2010), « Blood, urine, and sweat (BUS) study: monitoring and elimination of bioaccumulated toxic elements. ». Arch Environ Contam Toxicol., https://www.ncbi.nlm.nih.gov/pubmed/21057782

[ii] Crinnion WJ (2011), « Sauna as a valuable clinical tool for cardiovascular, autoimmune, toxicant- induced and other chronic health problems. », Altern Med Rev, https://www.ncbi.nlm.nih.gov/pubmed/21951023

[iii] Little P, Stuart B, Mullee M, Thomas T, Johnson S, Leydon G, Rabago D, Richards-Hall S, Williamson I, Yao G, Raftery J, Zhu S, Moore M; SNIFS Study Team (2016), « Effectiveness of steam inhalation and nasal irrigation for chronic or recurrent sinus symptoms in primary care: a pragmatic randomized controlled trial », CMAJ, https://www.ncbi.nlm.nih.gov/pubmed/27431306

[iv] Mahalingam S, Boominathan P (2016), « Effects of steam inhalation on voice quality-related acoustic measures » , Laryngoscope, https://www.ncbi.nlm.nih.gov/pubmed/26972609

[v] Scoon GS, Hopkins WG, Mayhew S, Cotter JD.(2007), « Effect of post-exercise sauna bathing on the endurance performance of competitive male runners », J Sci Med Sport, https://www.ncbi.nlm.nih.gov/pubmed/16877041

[vi] J. T. Selsby, S. Rother, S. Tsuda, O. Pracash, J. Quindry, and S. L. Dodd (2007), « Intermittent hyperthermia enhances skeletal muscle regrowth and attenuates oxidative damage following reloading », J Appl Physiol, https://www.ncbi.nlm.nih.gov/pubmed/17110516